THE LITTLE RED BOOK OF

DAD'S WISDOM

THE LITTLE RED BOOK OF
DAD'S WISDOM

Edited by Nick and Tony Lyons

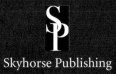

Skyhorse Publishing

Skyhorse Publishing books may be purchased in bulk at special discounts for
sales promotion, corporate gifts, fund-raising, or educational purposes. Special
editions can also be created to specifications. For details, contact the Special Sales
Department, Skyhorse Publishing, 307 West 36th Street, 11th Floor, New York,
NY 10018 or info@skyhorsepublishing.com.

Skyhorse® and Skyhorse Publishing® are registered trademarks of Skyhorse
Publishing, Inc.®, a Delaware corporation.

www.skyhorsepublishing.com

10 9 8 7 6 5 4 3 2 1

Library of Congress Cataloging-in-Publication Data is available on file.

ISBN: 978-1-61608-244-4

Printed in China

Contents

Introduction

"Fatherhood," says Annie Pigeon, "is a work in progress." And so it is. We know—we've been there together for nearly half a century. We've been connected, as father and son, for that long and on the way we've learned something about this endlessly fascinating relationship. And now that one of us is a rather new father and the other a grandfather, we're learning even more. We're sure of this: it is an astonishingly happy, challenging, various, and always evolving relationship, or set of relationships, this fatherhood.

In the beginning there are a father's expectations about any new child, his first or his fifth, and then his very personal feelings—often startlingly unexpected—about that new child. As father and child both grow older, it all keeps changing, and questions of love, admiration, delight, pride, duty, education, hopes, worries, discipline, confrontations, and so much more come into play, as the worlds of father and child change—and sometimes collide. The teenage years can be terrifically demanding for both. Sons are different from daughters. All children begin that most difficult transition into adulthood. Then grown children bring still other issues, as the family expands to include spouses and perhaps grandchildren, and sometimes even an opportunity (as happened for us) to be in business together (first, in our case, the son entered the father's business and now the opposite has happened). And when both father and children have grown older and perhaps more reflective, there are many moments for looking back over the arc of their lives, remembering, evaluating. "In progress," indeed. We've tried to include comments on all of these stages.

Great writers of all stripes, psychologists, eminent soldiers and statesmen, comedians, and a span of others have commented on the multi-faceted aspects of a father's relationship to his son or daughter, or to his or her feelings, and the words have been at times wise, at times hilarious, sometimes abrupt or raw, sometimes practical, and sometimes penetrating. And so much more.

We've enjoyed collecting some of the most interesting of these words and very much hope that you enjoy this diverse collection of observations by and about that common but so often misunderstood state known as fatherhood.

—Tony Lyons and Nick Lyons
Spring 2011

Being a dad is one of the oldest "professions"
around.
　　　　—MARCUS JACOB GOLDMAN,
　　　　THE JOY OF FATHERHOOD (2000)

THE LITTLE RED BOOK OF

DAD'S WISDOM

PART ONE

On Becoming a Father

We wanted you so badly. We loved you before
we saw you.
—PETER CAREY, "A LETTER TO OUR SON,"
THE CRANTA BOOK OF THE FAMILY (1995)

• • •

Some dads liken the impending birth of a child
to the beginning of a great journey.
—MARCUS JACOB GOLDMAN, *THE JOY OF
FATHERHOOD (2000)*

• •

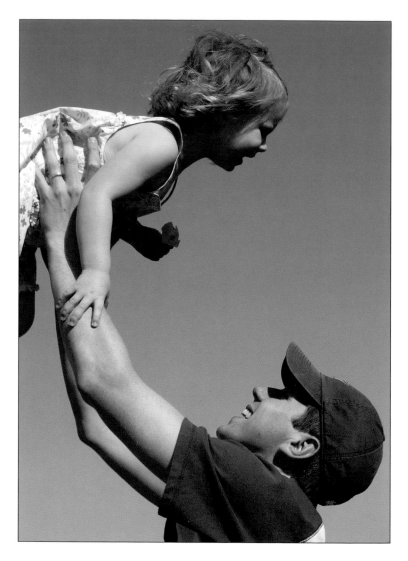

A baby is God's opinion that life should go on.
—CARL SANDBURG

• • •

For fathers-to-be, pregnancy also serves as a time
of profound transition: nine months of mental,
emotional, material, perhaps physical, and almost
certainly financial preparation to become a father.
—KEVIN OSBORN, *THE COMPLETE IDIOT'S GUIDE TO
FATHERHOOD (2000)*

• •

Arrange for paternity leave.
—ANNIE PIGEON, *DAD'S LITTLE INSTRUCTION BOOK*
(1995)

• • •

Many of us are not ready to be fathers when a
child comes.
—JOHN L. HART, *BECOMING A FATHER (1998)*

• •

I don't know any parents that look into the eyes
of a newborn baby and say, "How can we screw
this kid up?"
—RUSSELL BISHOP

• • •

On Becoming a Father

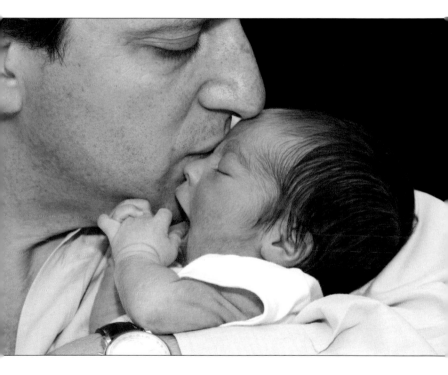

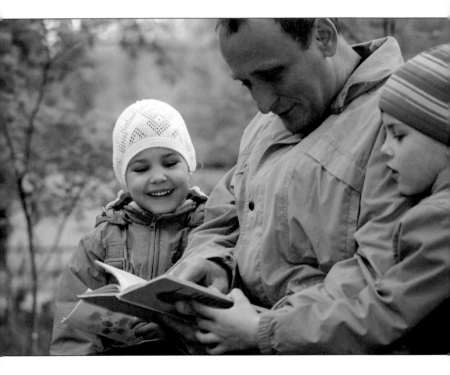

I felt something impossible for me to explain in
words. Then when they took her away, it hit me.
I got scared all over again and began to feel
giddy. Then it came to me—I was a father.
—NAT KING COLE

• •

When Charles first saw our child Mary, he said
all the proper things for a new father. He looked
upon the poor little red thing and blurted, "She's
more beautiful than the Brooklyn Bridge."
—HELEN HAYES

• • •

If you ever become a father, I think the strangest
and strongest sensation of your life will be hearing
for the first time the thin cry of your child.
—LAFCADIO HEARN (1850–1904)

• •

. . . when my son looks up at me and breaks into
his wonderful toothless smile, my eyes fill up
and I know that having him is the best thing I
will ever do.
—DAN GREENBERG

• • •

On Becoming a Father

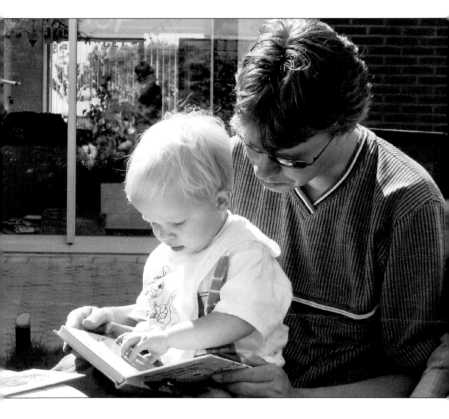

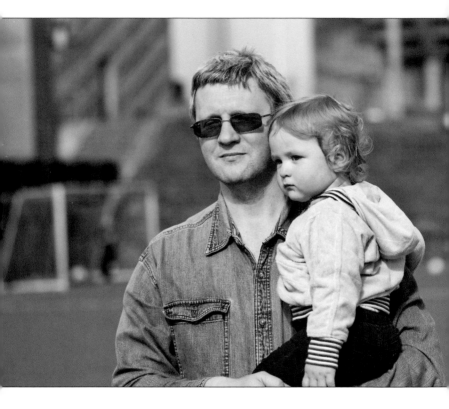

Men who have fought in the world's bloodiest wars . . . are apt to faint at the sight of a truly foul diaper.
—GARY D. CHRISTENSON

• •

Blessed indeed is the man who hears many gentle voices call him father!
—LYDIA M. CHILD

• • •

There are times when parenthood seems nothing but feeding the mouth that bites you.
—PETER DE VRIES

• •

A baby changes your dinner-party conversation
from politics to poops.
—MARCUS JACOB GOLDMAN, *THE JOY OF
FATHERHOOD (2000)*

• • •

The most common mistake in choosing a name
comes from forgetting the fiendish tortures that
kids inflict on other kids because of an unconventional
name, an unfortunate set of initials, or
a cute nickname that becomes less cute with
each passing year.
—PETER MAYLE, *HOW TO BE A PREGNANT FATHER*
(1995)

• •

She said, "There it is. I can see your baby's head." It was you. The tip of you, the top of you. You were a new country, a planet, a star seen for the first time.
—PETER CAREY, "A LETTER TO OUR SON," *THE GRANTA BOOK OF THE FAMILY (1995)*

• • •

. . . when my mother suggested that I be known by my middle name, Halsey, my father countered: "You might as well call him Abercrombie and completely do him in."
—WILLIAM PLUMMER, *WISHING MY FATHER WELL* (2000)

• •

"Is this kid beautiful, or is this kid beautiful?"
I always ask to hear the choices again, because
they sound so similar.
—PAUL REISER, *COUPLEHOOD (1994)*

• • •

Fatherhood was a mysterious state and didn't
seem to become any less so with time and familiarity.
At night, when I looked in on my sleeping
daughters, I would feel a deep sense of improbability
mingled with inadequacy.
—GEOFFREY NORMAN, *TWO FOR THE SUMMIT*
(2000)

• •

On Becoming a Father

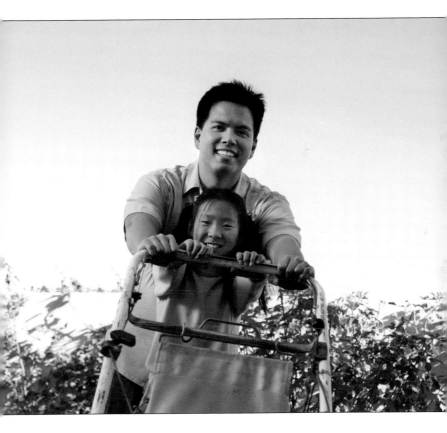

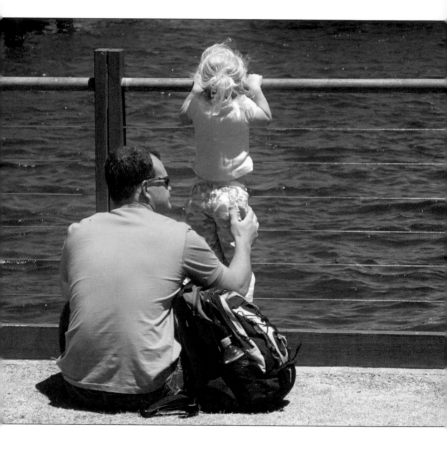

No man can possibly know what life means, what
the world means, what anything means, until he
has a child and loves it.
—LAFCADIO HEARN (1850–1904)

• • •

The child had every toy his father wanted.
—ROBERT C. WHITTEN

• •

When dealing with a two-year-old in the midst
of a tantrum, fathers need to be particularly
watchful about the tendency to need to feel
victorious.
—DR. KYLE PRUETT (QUOTED IN *DADS*,
JUNE/JULY 2000)

• • •

The best way to evaluate—and fine-tune—your
childproofing efforts is to get down on your
hands and knees and do a test run. Anything
you can reach, your child can reach.
—KEVIN OSBORN, *THE COMPLETE IDIOT'S GUIDE TO
FATHERHOOD (2000)*

• •

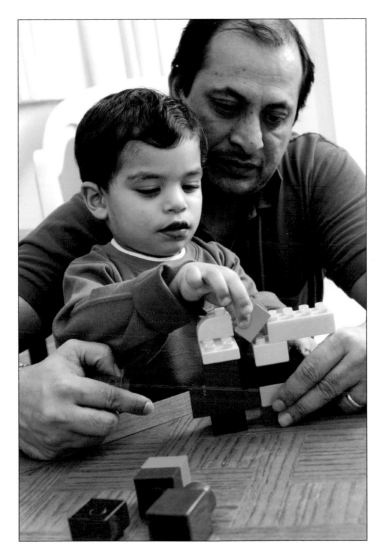

You look in the mirror and see the blurry image of two dads—one is tired, withered, drained, and pale, while the other is vibrant, enthusiastic, proud, and eager to meet the next challenge.
—MARCUS JACOB GOLDMAN, *THE JOY OF FATHERHOOD (2000)*

• • •

I used to think having a dog was adequate preparation for parenthood, but I'm told they're not exactly the same—pet ownership and child rearing.
—PAUL REISER, *COUPLEHOOD (1994)*

• •

. . . when I looked at you first I saw not your
mother and me, but your two grandfathers . . .
and, as my father, whom I loved a great deal, had
died the year before, I was moved to see that
here, in you, he was alive.
—PETER CAREY, "A LETTER TO OUR SON,"
THE GRANTA BOOK OF THE FAMILY (1995)

PART TWO

• • •

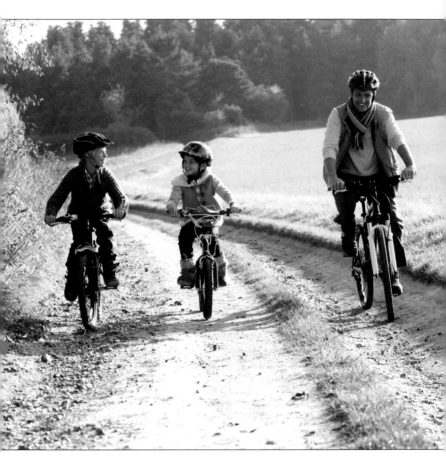

Being a Better Father

You know the only people who are always sure about the proper way to raise children? Those who've never had any.
—BILL COSBY, *FATHERHOOD*

• • •

It is easier for a father to have children than for children to have a real father.
—POPE JOHN XXIII

• •

I was the same kind of father as I was a harpist—I played by ear.
—HARPO MARX

• • •

Fathers, like mothers, are not born. Men grow into fathers—and fathering is a very important stage in their development.
—DAVID M. GOTTESMAN

• •

Fathers are pals nowadays because they don't
have the guts to be fathers.
—H. JACKSON BROWNE'S DAD, AS QUOTED IN
A FATHER'S BOOK OF WISDOM (1988)

• • •

If the statistics are true, by the time the average
American youngster is six, he will spend more
time watching television than he will spend talking
to his father in his lifetime.
—DR. JAMES DOBSON, *CHILDREN AT RISK*

• •

The most important thing a father can do for his children is to love their mother.
—THEODORE HESBURGH

• • •

To be a successful father . . . there's one absolute rule: when you have a kid, don't look at it for the first two years.
—ERNEST HEMINGWAY

• •

Hug.
—ANNIE PIGEON, *DAD'S LITTLE INSTRUCTION BOOK (1995)*

• • •

Being a Better Father

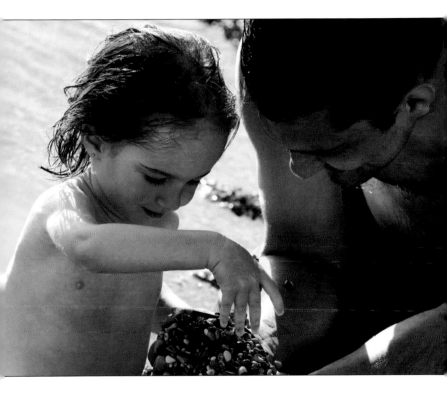

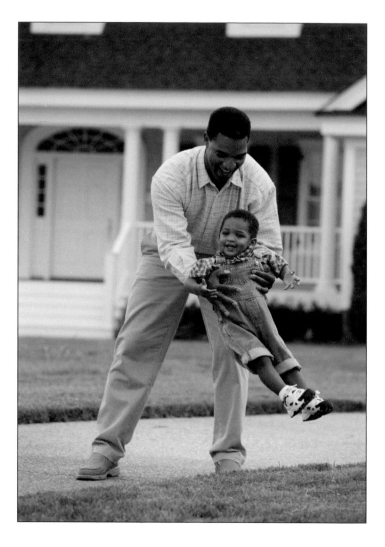

I cannot think of any need in childhood as strong
as the need for a father's protection.
—SIGMUND FREUD

• •

Ideally, they should give you a couple of "practice
kids" before you have any for real. Sort of
like bowling a few frames for free before you
start keeping score. Let you warm up.
—PAUL REISER, *COUPLEHOOD (1994)*

• • •

I have found the best way to give advice to your children is to find out what they want and then advise them to do it.
—HARRY S TRUMAN

• •

The father is always a Republican toward his son, and his mother's always a Democrat.
—ROBERT FROST

• • •

Unfortunately, children don't come already trained,
and whether we like it or not, they will sometimes
develop habits and attitudes which we need to
train them out of!
—IAN GRANT, *FATHERS WHO DARE TO WIN (1999)*

• •

My father didn't tell me how to live; he lived,
and let me watch him do it.
—CLARENCE KELLAND

• • •

I only wanted him to say he loved me.
—RUSSELL CHATHAM

• •

He that does not bring up his son to some honest
calling and employment brings him up to be
a thief.
—JEWISH PROVERB

• • •

A truly great man never puts away the simplicity
of a child.
—CONFUCIUS

• •

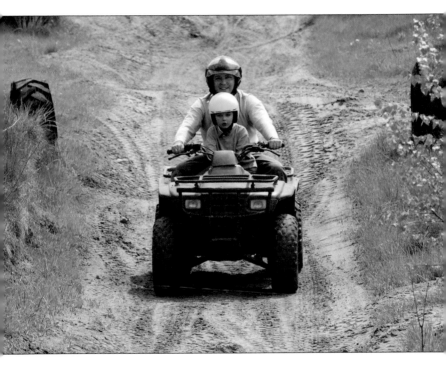

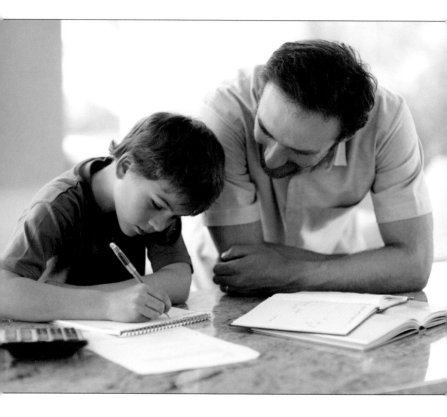

I am determined to be involved in my children's
lives because of my sorrow over my relationship
with my father.
—WILLIAM PLUMMER, *WISHING MY FATHER WELL*
(2000)

• • •

My son is seven years old. I am fifty-four. It has
taken me a great many years to reach that age.
I am more respected in the community, I am
stronger, I am more intelligent and I think I am
better than he is. I don't want to be his pal, I
want to be a father.
—CLIFTON FADIMAN

• •

My children give me the gift of stepping out
of the daily ordinariness into the father zone—a
place where my innate curiosity, sense of adventure,
and love of a weekend gets rediscovered.
—JEFF STONE, "CONFESSIONS OF A WEEKEND DAD"
(DADS, JUNE/JULY 2000)

• • •

Father of fathers, make me one,
A fit example for a son.
—DOUGLAS MALLOOCH

• •

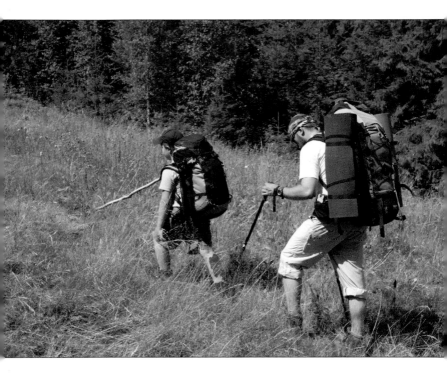

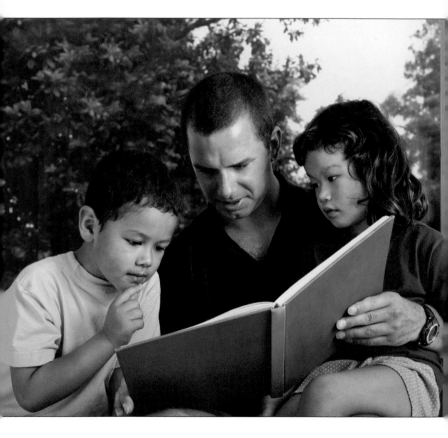

A young man asks an older musician, "How do I
get to Carnegie Hall?" To which the older man
answers, "Practice, my son, practice." You can say
the same for fatherhood.
—JEAN MARZOLLO, *FATHERS AND BABIES (1993)*

• • •

Parents should sit tall in the saddle and look
upon their troops with a noble and benevolent
and extremely nearsighted gaze.
—GARRISON KEILLOR

• •

Let us teach them not only to do virtuously,
but to excel. To excel they must be taught to be
steady, active, and industrious.
—JOHN ADAMS, TO HIS WIFE ABIGAIL

• • •

By profession I am a soldier and take great pride
in that fact, but I am also prouder, infinitely
prouder, to be a father. A soldier destroys in order
to build; the father only builds, never destroys.
—DOUGLAS MACARTHUR, *REMINISCENCES (1964)*

• •

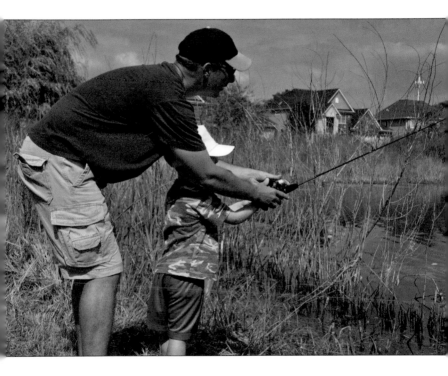

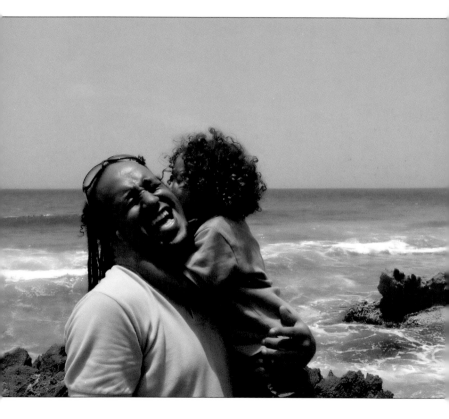

It takes time to be a good father. It takes effort—trying,
failing, and trying again.
—TIM HANSEL, AS QUOTED IN *DAD'S APPRECIATION
BOOK* OF *WIT AND WISDOM (1996)*

• • •

Fathers, provoke not your children to anger, lest
they be discouraged.
—*THE HOLY BIBLE,* COLOSSIANS 3:20

• •

One father is more than a hundred school-masters.
—GEORGE HERBERT (1593–1633)

• • •

Govern a family as you would cook a small fish—very gently.
—CHINESE PROVERB

• •

I grew up thinking my parents knew everything. I'm sure they didn't, but at least they were smart enough to fake it. I don't even know how to do that yet.
—PAUL REISER, *COUPLEHOOD (1994)*

• • •

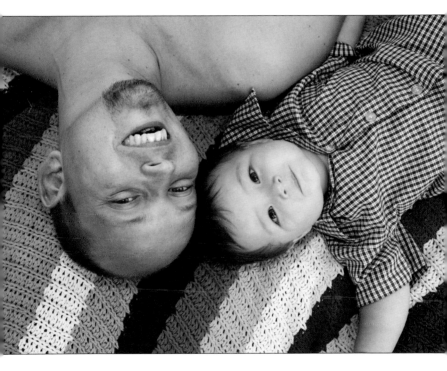

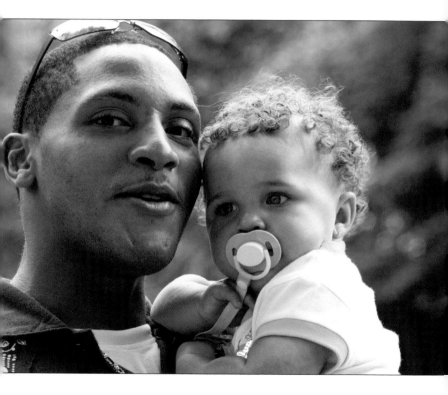

To show a child what once delighted you, to find
the child's delight added to your own so that
there is now a double delight seen in the glow of
trust and affection, this is happiness.
—J. B. PRIESTLEY (1894–1984)

• •

Fatherhood was full-time work for Dad. When I
was about ten, I took up the clarinet. Instead of
buying me a metronome and sending me off to a
soundproof room to squeak my way through the
scales, he sat with me and beat time against the
arm of his chair with his pipe.
—WILLIAM G. TAPPLY, *SPORTSMAN'S LEGACY (1993)*

• • •

Never raise your hand to your child; it leaves
your midsection unprotected.
—ROBERT ORBEN

• •

The lone father is not a strong father. Fathering
is a difficult and perilous journey and is done
well with the help of other men.
—JOHN L. HART, *BECOMING A FATHER (1998)*

• • •

Raising children is part joy and part guerrilla
warfare.
—ED ASNER

• •

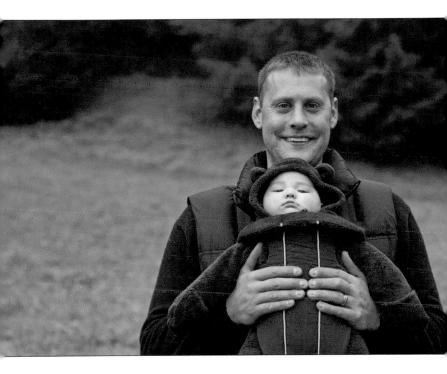

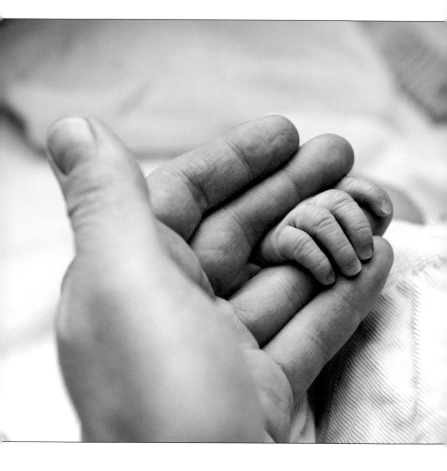

The American father . . . passes his life entirely on
Wall Street and communicates with his family
once a month by means of a telegram in cipher.
—OSCAR WILDE

• • •

The fundamental defect of fathers is that they
want their children to be a credit to them.
—BERTRAND RUSSELL

• •

If the new American father feels bewildered and
even defeated, let him take comfort from the fact
that whatever he does in any fathering situation
has a fifty percent chance of being right.
—BILL COSBY

• • •

No, you can't charge them rent when they're still
in grade school.
—ANNIE PIGEON, *DAD'S LITTLE INSTRUCTION
BOOK (1995)*

• •

Raising a child on a steady diet of "I am the
center of the universe" is generally quite harmful.
Your child is not the center of the universe
and never will be.
—IAN GRANT, *FATHERS WHO DARE TO WIN (1999)*

• • •

A father is a man who is always learning to love.
He knows that his love must grow and change
because his children change.
—TIM HANSEL, AS QUOTED IN *DAD'S APPRECIATION
BOOK OF WIT AND WISDOM (1996)*

• •

Mostly you just have to keep plugging and keep
loving—and hoping that your child forgives you
according to how you loved him, judged him,
forgave him, and stood watching over him as he
slept, year after year.
—BEN STEIN, "MISTAKES OF THE FATHER"
(DADS, JUNE/JULY 2000)

PART THREE

• • •

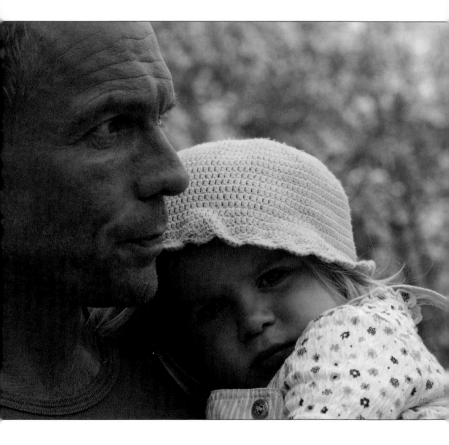

Fathers and Daughters

The lucky man has a daughter as his first child.
—SPANISH PROVERB (QUOTED IN *TWO FOR THE
SUMMIT,* GEOFFREY NORMAN, 2000)

• • •

When he saw his daughters happy he knew that
he had done well.
—HONORE DE BALZAC, *PERE GORlOT*

• •

A girl's father is the first man in her life, and
probably the most influential.
—DAVID JEREMIAH (QUOTED IN *FATHERS WHO DARE
TO WIN* BY IAN GRANT, 1999)

• • •

To her the name of father was another name for
love.
—FANNY FERN

• •

Fathers and Daughters

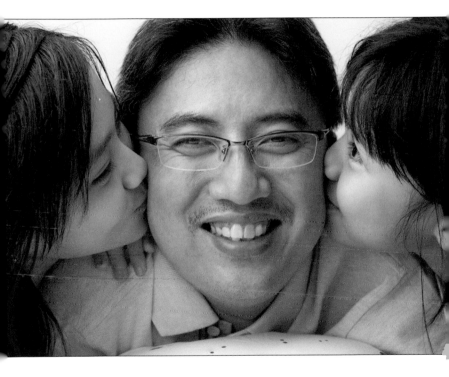

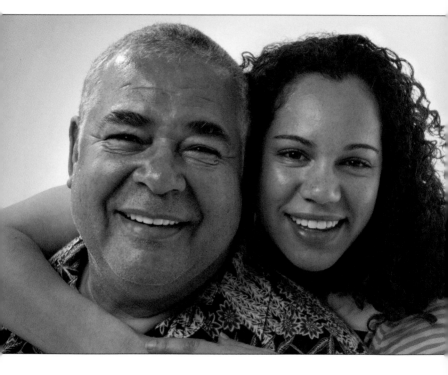

Daughters, I think, are always easier for fathers.
I don't know why.
—WILLIAM PLUMMER, *WISHING MY FATHER
WELL (2000)*

• • •

It no longer bothers me that I may be constantly
searching for father figures; by this time, I have
found several and dearly enjoyed knowing
them all.
—ALICE WALKER

• •

She got the good looks from her father—he's a
plastic surgeon.
—GROUCHO MARX

• • •

A father is always making his baby into a little
woman. And when she is a woman he turns her
back again.
—ENID BAGNOLD

• •

I didn't have to do much, if anything, to rate a
hug from one of my girls.
—GEOFFREY NORMAN, *TWO FOR THE
SUMMIT (2000)*

• • •

Rose was like her father for all the world . . . she
was always quoting her father—in fact, we used
to call her "Father says."
—A CHILDHOOD FRIEND OF ROSE KENNEDY,
QUOTED IN *ROSE* BY GAIL CAMERON (1971)

• •

His sole pleasure was to gratify his daughters'
whims . . . Goriot raised his daughters to the rank
of angels, and so of necessity above himself.
—HONORE DE BALZAC, *PERE GORIOT*

• • •

Someday I'll be his student too—then I won't be
his daughter.
—LARA (AGE 4) OF HER FATHER, A TEACHER

• •

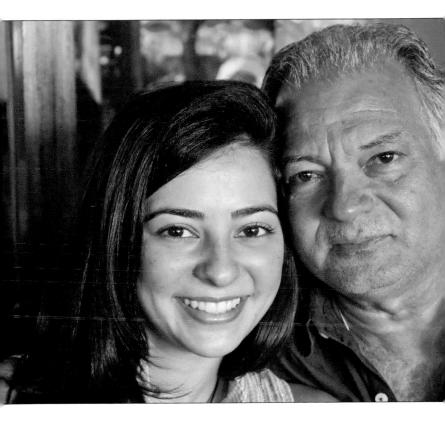

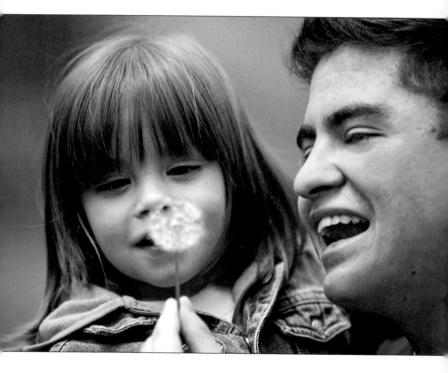

Nothing is dearer to an old father than a daughter.
Sons have spirits of higher pitch, but they are
not given to fondness.
—EURIPIDES

• • •

It isn't that I'm a weak father, it's just that she's a
strong daughter.
—HENRY FONDA

• •

When a girl reaches adolescence, she looks to
her father for approval and love.
—IAN GRANT, *FATHERS WIIO DARE TO WIN (1999)*

• • •

I can run the country or control Alice [his
daughter]. I can't do both.
—THEODORE ROOSEVELT

• •

. . . you want your daughters to adore you . . .
without reservation and without my doing anything
to deserve it, for the sheer accidental reason
that I was the only man in their young lives.
—GEOFFREY NORMAN, *TWO FOR THE
SUMMIT (2000)*

• • •

Fathers and Daughters

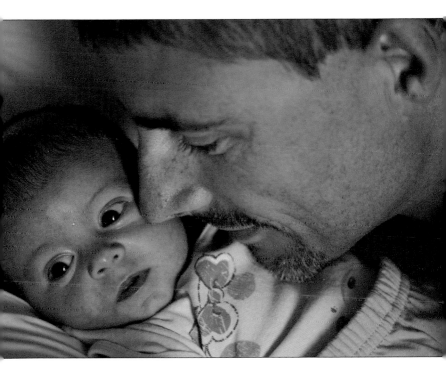

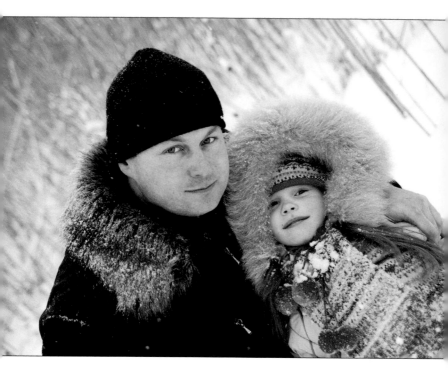

Many a man wishes he were strong enough to
tear a telephone book in half—especially if he
has a teenage daughter.
—GUY LOMBARDO

• •

You didn't want to boast that you have scared
as feckless a father as I am into chronic sleeplessness.
—ROBERT FROST, TO HIS DAUGHTER LESLEY,
QUOTED IN *THE BOOK* OF *FATHER'S WISDOM,* ED.
EDWARD HOFFMAN (1997)

• • •

Things not to worry about:
–Don't worry about popular opinion
–Don't worry about dolls
–Don't worry about the past
—F. SCOTT FITZGERALD, TO HIS DAUGHTER SCOTTIE

• •

True maturity is only reached when a man realizes
he has become a father figure to his daughters'
girlfriends—and he accepts it.
—LARRY MCMURTRY

• • •

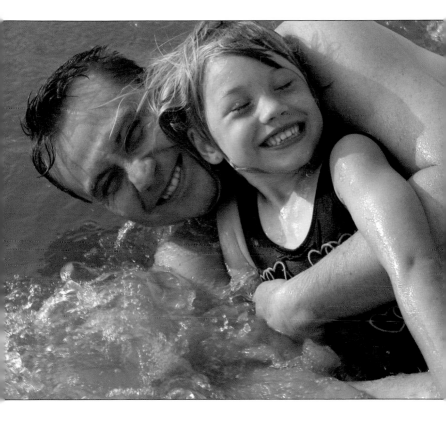

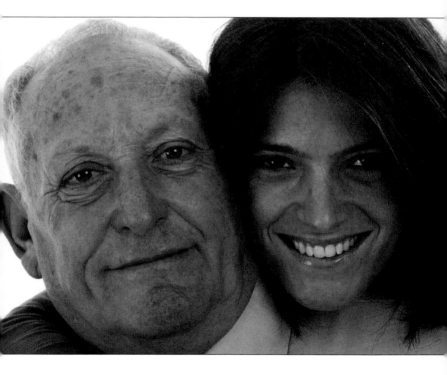

Tell me, my daughters,
Since now we will divest us
Both of rule,
Interest of territory, cares of State,
Which of you shall we say doth love us most?
— KING LEAR TO HIS THREE DAUGHTERS, IN
KING LEAR BY WILLIAM SHAKESPEARE

• •

All right, I'll give you fifty dollars to help pay
your expenses for a couple of weeks, until you
recover from this madness, but that's the last
penny you'll get from me until you do something
respectable.
—THOMAS HEPBURN, TO HIS DAUGHTER
KATHARINE HEPBURN (QUOTED IN *FATHER KNEW
BEST, 1997)*

• • •

You mustn't get aggravated when your old dad
calls you his baby, because he always will think
of you as just that—no matter how old or big
you may get.
—HARRY S TRUMAN, TO HIS DAUGHTER MARGARET

• •

It doesn't matter who my father was; it matters
who I remember he was.
—ANNE SEXTON

• • •

We are so young when we marry—what do we
know of the world or of men? Our fathers ought
to think for us.
—DELPHINE TO HER FATHER IN *PERE GORIOT* BY
HONORE DE BALZAC

• •

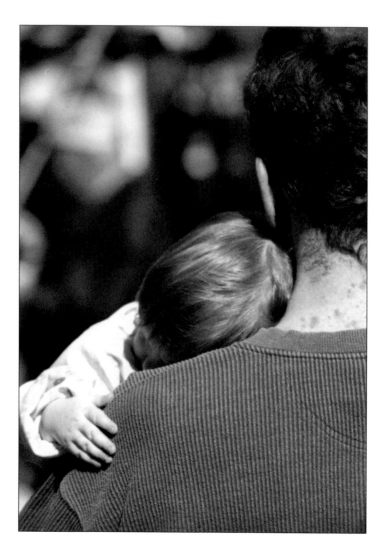

PART FOUR

Fathers and Sons

Like father, like son.
—ANONYMOUS

• • •

Build me a son, O Lord, who will be strong
enough to know when he is weak, and brave
enough to face himself when he is afraid, one
who will be proud and unbending in honest defeat,
and humble and gentle in victory.
—DOUGLAS MCARTHUR, "A FATHER'S PRAYER"

• •

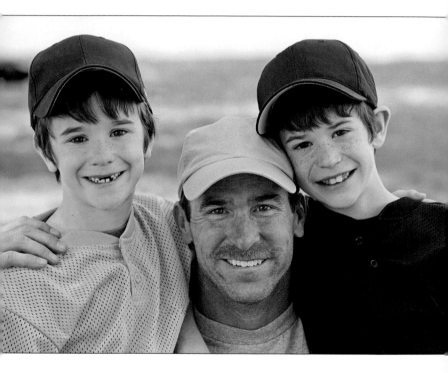

A boy, by the age of three years, senses that his
destiny is to be a man, so he watches his father
particularly—his interests, manner, speech,
pleasures, his attitude toward work . . .
—BENJAMIN SPOCK AND MICHAEL B. ROTHENBERG,
DR. SPOCK'S BABY AND CHILD CARE (1992)

• • •

'Tis a happy thing to be a father unto many sons.
—WILLIAM SHAKESPEARE, *HENRY VI*

• •

I like my boy . . . and his utter inability to conceive
why I should not leave all my nonsense,
business, and writing and come to tie up his toy
horse . . .
—RALPH WALDO EMERSON

• • •

I enclose $1.00. Spend it liberally, generously,
carefully, judiciously, sensibly. Get from it pleasure,
wisdom, health, and experience.
—EDWARD FITZGERALD, TO HIS SON
F. SCOTT FITZGERALD (QUOTED IN *FATHER
KNEW BEST,* 1997)

• •

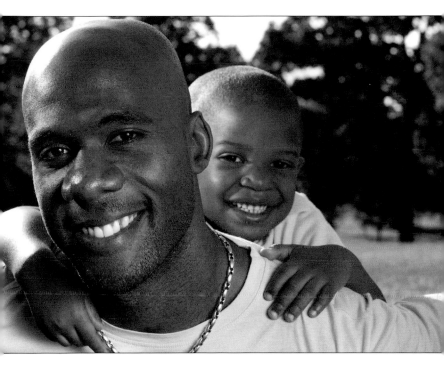

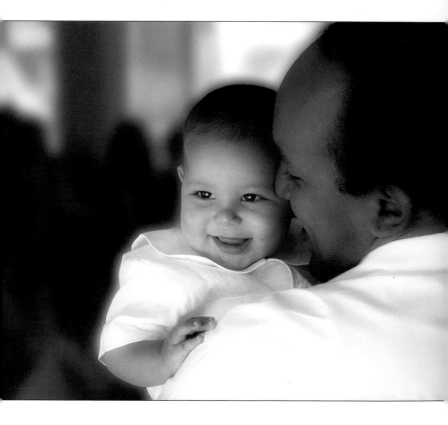

I never got along with my dad. Kids used to
come up to me and say, "My dad can beat up
your dad." I'd say, "Yeah? When?"
—BILL HICKS

• • •

Like so much else between fathers and sons,
playing catch was tender and tense at the same
time.
—DONALD HALL

• •

The son hopes the father will talk to him. What he really hopes is that the suit of armor that is his father will teeter once or twice, creak, and fall over . . .
—CHARLES GAINES

• • •

John Elway is a great football player. He used to be my son. Now I'm his father.
—JACK ELWAY

• •

If my own son, who is now ten months, came to me and said, "You promised to pay for my tuition at Harvard; how about giving me $50,000 instead to start a little business," I might think that was a good idea.
—WILLIAM BENNETT

• • •

I cheat my boys every chance I get. It makes 'em sharp.
—WILLIAM ROCKEFELLER (JOHN D.'S FATHER)

• •

His father watched him across the gulf of years
and pathos which always divide a father from
his son.
—JOHN MARQUAND

• • •

If the relationship of father to son could really be
reduced to biology, the earth would blaze with
the glory of fathers and sons.
—JAMES BALDWIN

• •

Fathers and Sons

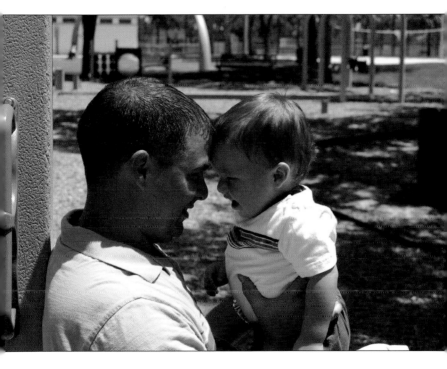

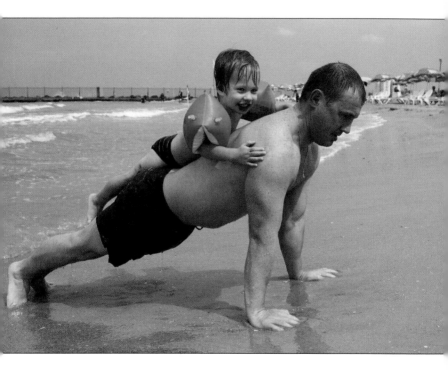

My father was frightened of his father, I was frightened of my father, and I am damned well going to see to it that my children are frightened of me.
—KING GEORGE V

• • •

A father is a man who expects his son to be as good a man as he meant to be.
—FRANK A. CLARK

• •

There is nothing more common, more natural,
than for fathers and sons to be strangers to each other.
—MICHAEL IGNATIEFF, "AUGUST IN MY
FATHER'S HOUSE," *THE GRANTA BOOK OF
THE FAMILY (1995)*

• • •

A father follows the course of his son's life and
notes many things of which he has not the privilege
to speak.
—WILLIAM CARLOS WILLIAMS, *THE SELECTED
LETTERS OF WILLIAM CARLOS WILLIAMS (1957)*

• •

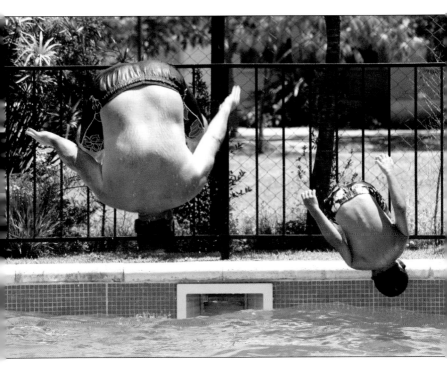

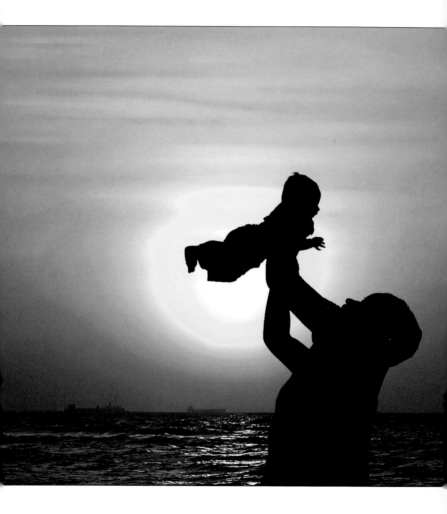

The land of my fathers. My fathers can have it.
—DYLAN THOMAS, ON WALES

• • •

. . . it's easy to wind back thirty or forty years to
other times when Dad and I have been together
in the woods beside a stream. It never really
mattered where we were or whether we had
caught many trout or found a lot of birds. Time
and place were irrelevant as long as we shared them.
—WILLIAM C. TAPPLY, *SPORTSMAN'S LEGACY (1993)*

• •

I didn't know the full facts of life until I was seventeen.
My father never talked about his work.
—MARTIN FREUD, SON OF SIGMUND FREUD

• • •

My father would have enjoyed what you have so
generously said of me—and my mother would
have believed it.
—LYNDON B. JOHNSON

• •

Perhaps host and guest is really the happiest
relation for father and son.
—EVELYN WAUGH

• • •

Baseball is fathers and sons playing catch, lazy
and murderous, wild and controlled, the profound
archaic song of birth, growth, age, and
death.
—DONALD HALL

• •

For rarely are sons similar to their fathers: most
are worse, and few are better . . .
—HOMER

• • •

There must always be a struggle between a
father and son, while one aims at power and the
other at independence.
—SAMUEL JOHNSON

• •

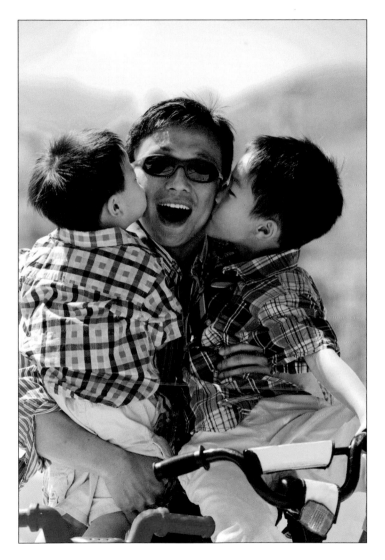

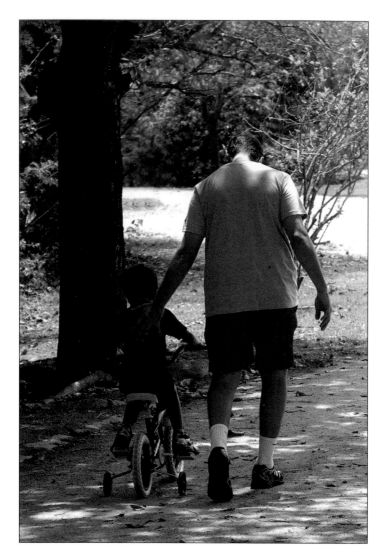

We think of our Fathers Fools, so wise we grow;
Our wiser Sons, no doubt, will think us so.
—ALEXANDER POPE

• • •

The father who does not teach his son his duties
is equally guilty with the son who neglects them.
— CONFUCIUS

• •

I distrust any man who claims to have had a
continuous friendship with his father. How did
he get from fourteen to twenty-six?
—VERLYN KUNKENBORG

• • •

Fathers send their sons to college either because
they went to college or because they didn't.
—L. L. HENDERSON

• •

Any boy your age who disobeys his mother, or
worries her, or is disrespectful to her—such a
boy is a poor, shabby fellow; and, if you know
such boys, you ought to cut their acquaintance.
—HERMAN MELVILLE, TO HIS SON MALCOLM

• • •

I am delighted to have you play football. I believe
in rough, manly sports. But I do not believe
in them if they degenerate into the sole end of
anyone's existence.
—THEODORE ROOSEVELT, TO HIS SON THEODORE
ROOSEVELT, JR.

• •

I think the saddest day of my life was when I realized
I could beat my dad at most things, and
Bart experienced that at the age of four.
—HOMER J. SIMPSON

• • •

If the past cannot teach the present, and the father
cannot teach the son, then history need not
have bothered to go on, and the world has wasted
a great deal of time.
—RUSSELL HOBAN

• •

Fathers and Sons

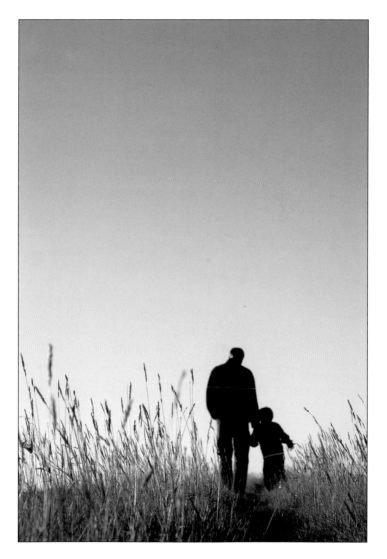

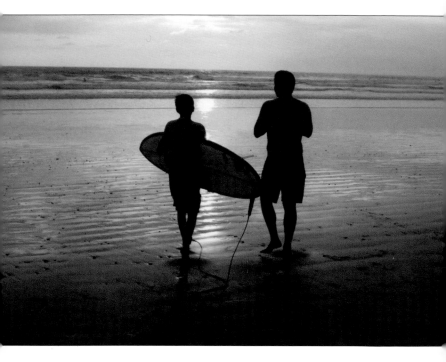

Never fret for an only son. The idea of failure will
never occur to him.
—GEORGE BERNARD SHAW

• • •

You don't raise heroes, you raise sons. And if you
treat them like sons, they'll turn out to be heroes
if it's just in your own eyes.
—WALTER M. SCHIRRA, SR.

• •

[It was like] dealing with Dad—all give and no take.
—JOHN F. KENNEDY, AFTER MEETING
WITH KHRUSHCHEV

• • •

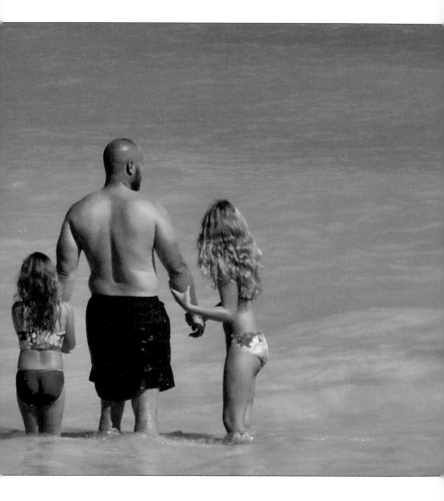

PART FIVE

Father Knows Best

What I learned is that if I don't know something,
I just shrug my shoulders and admit it.
Doctors don't know everything. Neither do teachers.
Or dads.
—FRANK MCCOURT (QUOTED IN *DADS*,
JUNE/JULY 2000)

• • •

The important thing, I learned from my father,
was to find your own bone and sink your teeth
in it.
—WILLIAM PLUMMER, *WISHING MY
FATHER WELL* (2000)

• •

My father told me there's no difference between
a black snake and a white snake. They both bite.
—THURGOOD MARSHALL

• • •

Can't you practice the drums quietly?
—BRUCE LANSKY AND K. L. JONES, *DADS SAY THE*
DUMBEST THINGS (1989)

• •

Father Knows Best

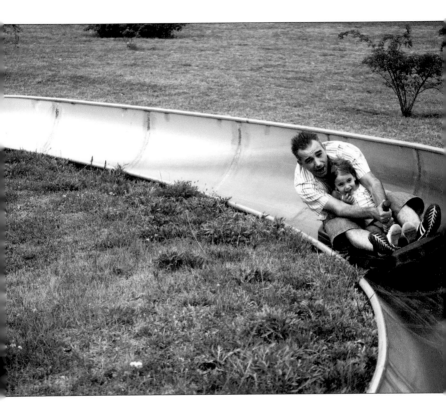

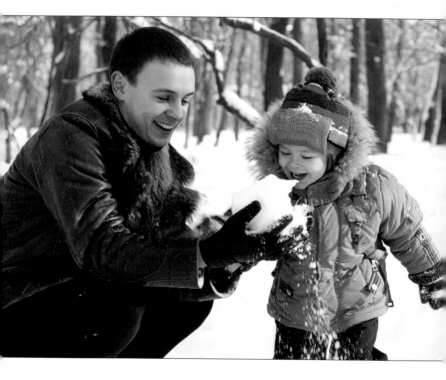

My father instilled in me the attitude of prevailing.
If there's a challenge, go for it. If there's a
wall to break down, break it down.
—DONNY OSMOND

• • •

Manual labor to my father was not only good
and decent for its own sake but, as he was given
to saying, it straightened out one's thoughts.
—MARY ELLEN CHASE

• •

Always obey your parents when they are present.
—MARK TWAIN

• • •

My father used to say, "Let them see you and not the suit. That should be secondary."
—CARY GRANT

• •

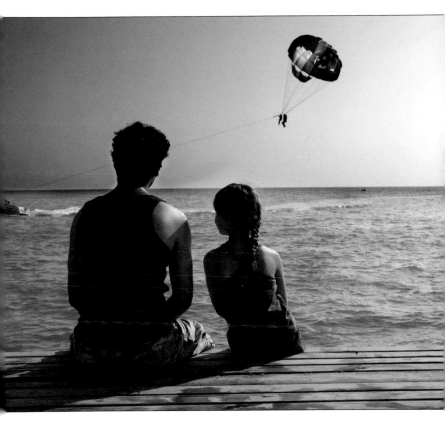

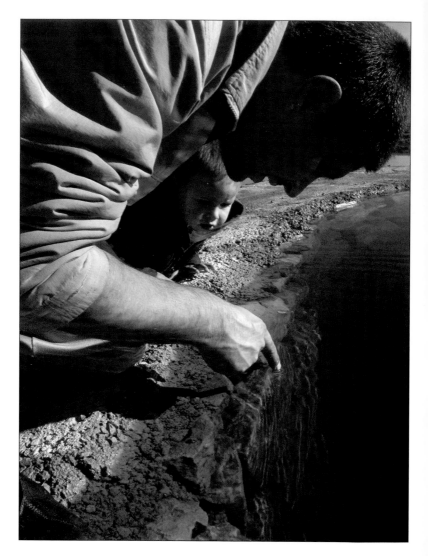

My father had always said there are four things a
child needs: plenty of love, nourishing food, regular
sleep, and lots of soap and water. After that,
what he needs most is some intelligent neglect.
—IVY BAKER PRIEST

• • •

My father, who was in politics, told me to remain
a bit mysterious. It makes people wonder about
you, draws them to you as we are all drawn to a mystery.
—JOE MILLS, QUOTED IN *FROM FATHER TO SON,* BY
ALLEN APPEL (1993)

• •

My father was very sure about certain matters
pertaining to the universe. To him, all good
things—trout as well as eternal salvation—come
by grace and grace comes by art, and art does
not come easy.
—NORMAN MACLEAN, *A RIVER RUNS
THROUGH IT (1976)*

• • •

Moss Hart . . . once announced that in dealing
with his children he kept one thing in mind:
"We're bigger than they are, and it's our house."
—JEAN KERR, *PLEASE DON'T EAT THE DAISIES*

• •

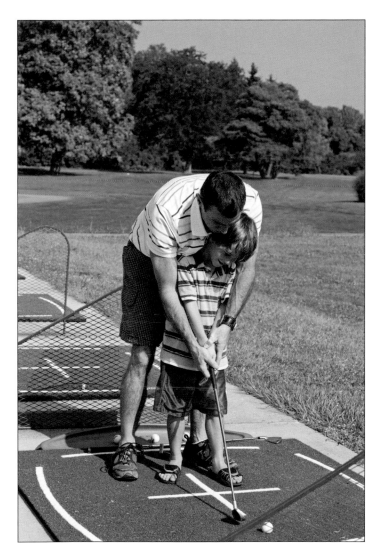

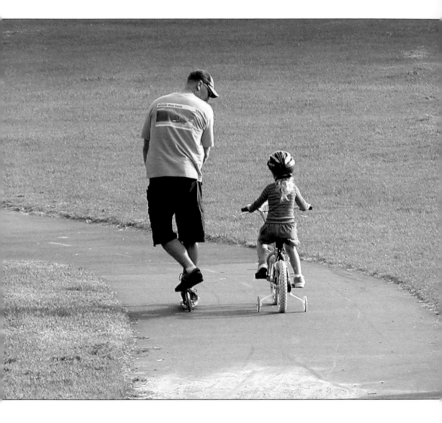

From my mother I learned to make pie crusts
and to iron shirts. From my father I learned to
catnap and to tell time without a watch.
—VERLYN KLINKENBORG

• • •

My father used to say that we must surrender
our youth to purchase wisdom. What he never
told me was how badly we get cheated on the
exchange rate.
—MORRIS WEST

• •

A birthday is a good time to begin anew: throwing
away the old habits, as you would old clothes,
and never putting them on again.
—BRONSON ALCOTT, TO HIS DAUGHTER ANNA

• • •

You're not a man until your father says you're
a man.
—BURT REYNOLDS

• •

Father taught us that opportunity and responsibility
go hand in hand. I think we all act on that
principle; on the basic human impulse that makes
a man want to make the best of what's in him
and what's been given him.
—LAURENCE ROCKEFELLER

• • •

Above all, I would teach him to tell the truth . . .
Truth-telling, I have found, is the key to responsible
citizenship. The thousands of criminals I
have seen in forty years of law enforcement have
had one thing in common: Every single one was
a liar.
—J. EDGAR HOOVER, "WHAT I WOULD
TELL A SON"

• •

My father gave me these hints on speech-making:
"Be sincere . . . be brief . . . be seated."
—JAMES ROOSEVELT

• • •

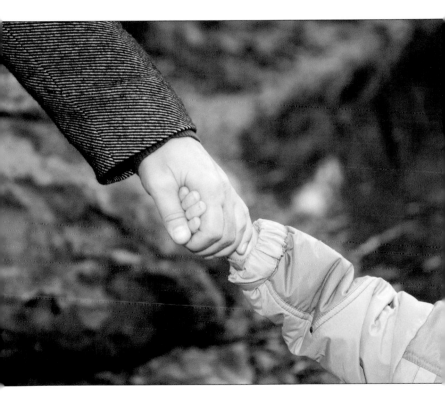

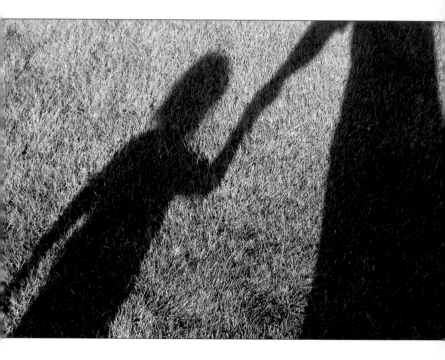

My father gave me the greatest gift anyone could
give another person. He believed in me.
—JIM VALVANO

• •

As a Scot and a Presbyterian, my father believed
that man by nature was a mess and had fallen
from an original state of grace. Somehow, I early
developed the notion that he had done this by
falling from a tree.
—NORMAN MACLEAN, *A RIVER RUNS
THROUGH IT (1976)*

• • •

My father taught me to be independent and
cocky, and free thinking, but he could not stand
it if I disagreed with him.
—SARA MAITLAND

• •

Mind you, don't go looking for fights, but if you
find yourself in one, make damn sure you win.
—CLYDE MORRISON, TO HIS SON JOHN WAYNE
(QUOTED IN *FATHER KNEW BEST,* 1997*)*

• • •

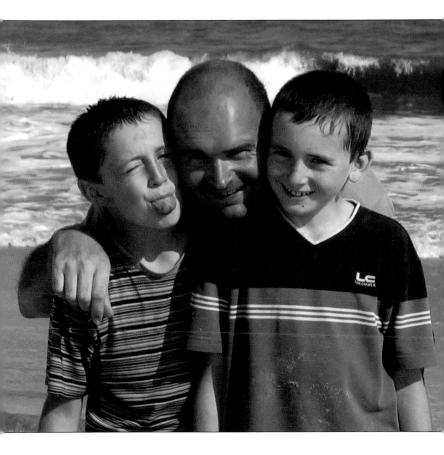

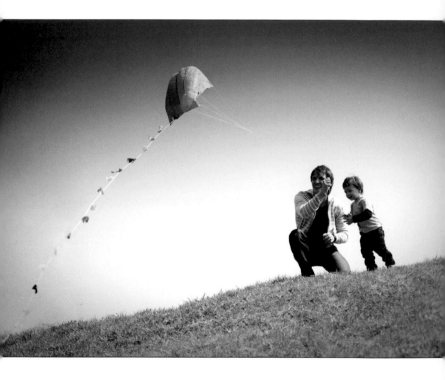

My father taught me to work; he did not teach
me to love it.
—ABRAHAM LINCOLN

• •

When I was a kid, I used to imagine animals
running under my bed. I told my dad, and he
solved the problem quickly. He cut the legs off
my bed.
—LOU BROCK

• • •

I hope when you grow up you will dedicate your life to trying to work out plans to make people happy instead of making them miserable, as war does today.
—JOSEPH P. KENNEDY, TO HIS SON EDWARD, AGE 8 (1946)

• •

This above all: to thine own self be true, and it must follow, as the night the day, thou canst not then be false to any man.
—POLONIUS, TO HIS SON LAERTES, IN *HAMLET* BY WILLIAM SHAKESPEARE

• • •

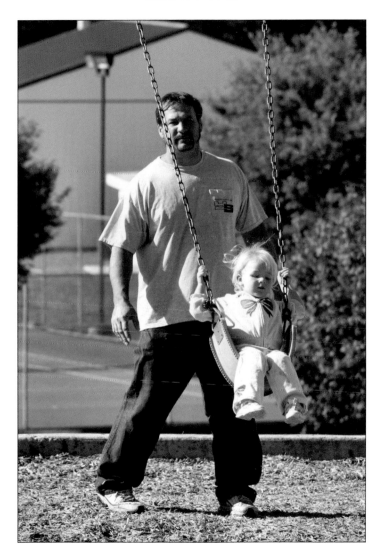

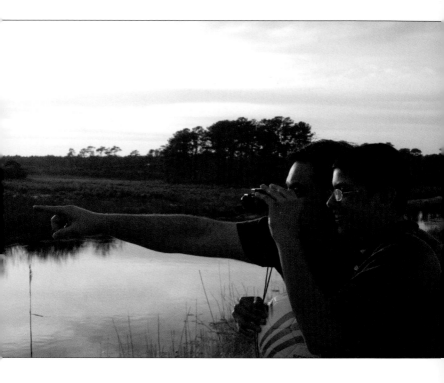

My dad has always taught me these words: care
and share.
—TIGER WOODS

• •

Dad often said, "A man that doesn't pick up a
penny that's laying on the ground won't ever
amount to much."
—RIC ANDERSON, QUOTED IN *FROM FATHER TO
SON,* BY ALLEN APPEL (1993)

• • •

As you journey through [life], you will encounter
all sorts of these nasty little upsets, and you will
either learn to adjust yourself to them or gradually
go nuts.
—GROUCHO MARX, TO HIS SON ARTHUR

• •

I have never smoked. I have my father to thank
for that.
—JIMMY CARTER, *EVERYTHING TO GAIN (1987)*

• • •

Father Knows Best

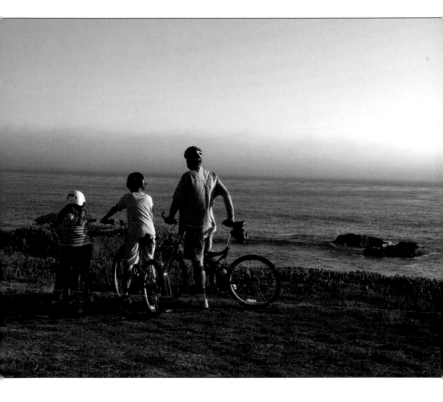

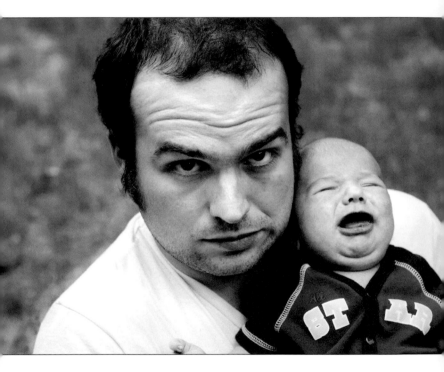

So subtle were his teachings, though, that I never
knew they were his until I became a parent myself
and saw my father in me as I began to shape
my own children's lives.
—KENNETH BARRETT

• •

A man's children and his garden both reflect
the amount of weeding done during the growing
season.
—AUTHOR UNKNOWN

• • •

The best advice ever given me was from my father.
When I was a little girl, he told me, "Don't
spend anything unless you have to."
—DINAH SHORE

• •

I expect I must, in part, have developed my notion
of character from watching my father struggle
against the mesquite.
—LARRY MCMURTRY, *WALTER BENJAMIN AT THE
DAIRY QUEEN (1999)*

• • •

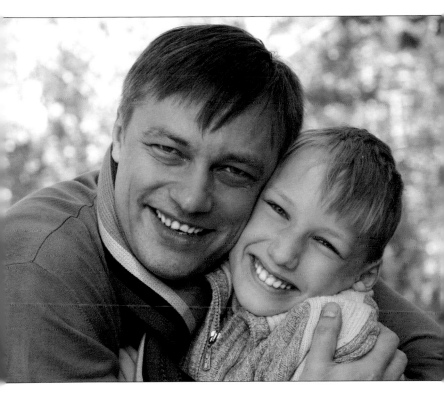

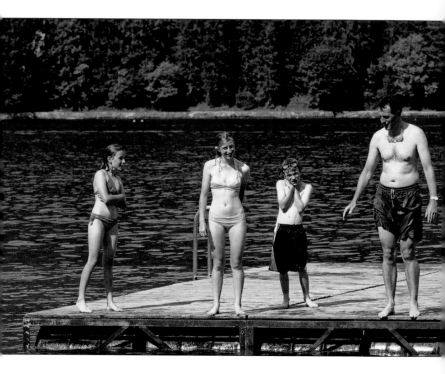

. . . and while I want you to keep looking well, I
think that if you spent a little more time picking
up your clothes instead of leaving them on
the floor, it wouldn't be necessary to have them
pressed so often.
—JOSEPH P. KENNEDY, TO HIS SON JACK,
AGE 14 (1932)

• •

Neither a borrower nor a lender be;
For loan oft loses both itself
And friend,
And borrowing dulls the edge of husbandry.
—POLONIUS, TO HIS SON LAERTES IN *HAMLET* BY
WILLIAM SHAKESPEARE

• • •

My father taught me that the only way you can
make good at anything is to practice, and then
practice some more.
—PETE ROSE

• •

What a father says to his children is not heard by
the world; but it will be heard by posterity.
—JEAN PAUL RICHTER

• • •

PART SIX

A Hard Profession

We are given children to test us and make us
more spiritual.
—GEORGE F. WILL

• • •

How children survive being brought up amazes
me.
—MALCOLM S. FORBES

• •

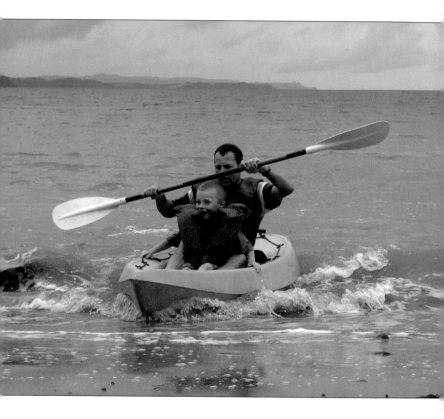

Like any father, I have moments when I wonder
whether I belong to the children or they belong
to me.
—BOB HOPE

• • •

A father is a guy who has snapshots in his wallet
where his money used to be.
—AUTHOR UNKNOWN

• •

I feel really lucky that my children have inherited
all good traits: looks, charm, wisdom, and objectivity.
—ROBERT SCOTELLARO

• • •

You don't have to deserve your mother's love.
You have to deserve your father's.
—ROBERT FROST

• •

Remember: fatherhood is a work in progress.
—ANNIE PIGEON, *DAD'S LITTLE
INSTRUCTION BOOK (1995)*

• • •

That is the thankless position of the father in
the family—the provider for all, and the enemy
of all.
—J. AUGUST STRINDBERG

• •

Every parent is at some time the father of the
unreturned prodigal, with nothing to do but keep
his house open to hope.
—JOHN CIARDI

• • •

My father sat up all night by the open casket
with the body of his son . . . . He smoked and he
drank and he whispered to his son, he made him
promises . . .
—JIM FERGUS, "MY FATHER'S SON,"
IN *FATHERS AND SONS*, ED. DAVID SEYBOLD (1992)

• •

There is no good father, that's the rule. Don't lay
the blame on men but on the bond of paternity,
which is rotten. To beget children, nothing better;
to have them, what iniquity!
—JEAN-PAUL SARTRE

• • •

Today, while the titular head of the family may
still be the father, everyone knows that he is little
more than chairman, at most, of the entertainment
committee.
—ASHLEY MONTAGU

• •

A Hard Profession

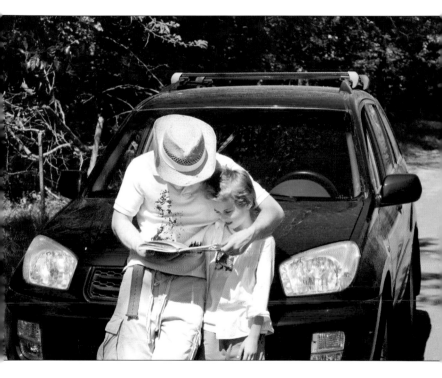

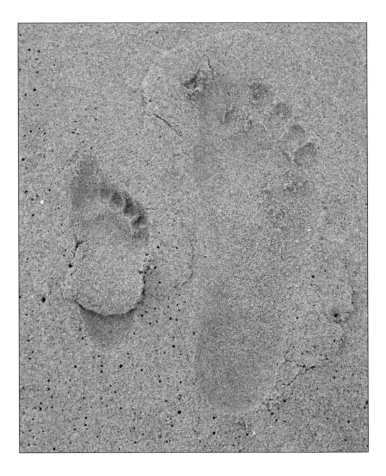

Insanity is hereditary; you can get it from your
children.
—SAM LEVENSON

• • •

My father the banker would shudder to see
In the back of his bank a painter to be.
—PAUL CEZANNE

• •

Children need models rather than critics.
—JOSEPH JOUBERT

• • •

I grew up to have my father's looks—my father's
speech patterns—my father's posture—my father's
walk—my father's opinions and my
mother's contempt for my father.
—JULES FEIFFER

• •

Every child . . . has a right to privacy as to its own
doings and its own affairs as much as if it were
its own father.
—G. B. SHAW

• • •

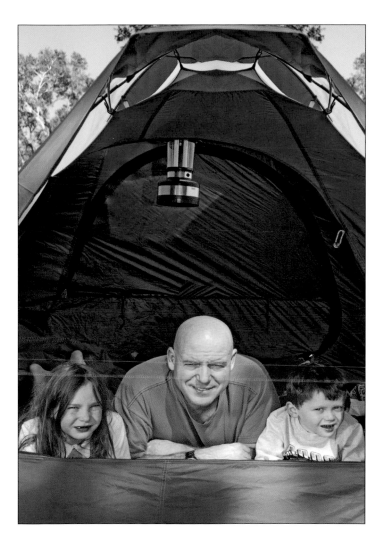

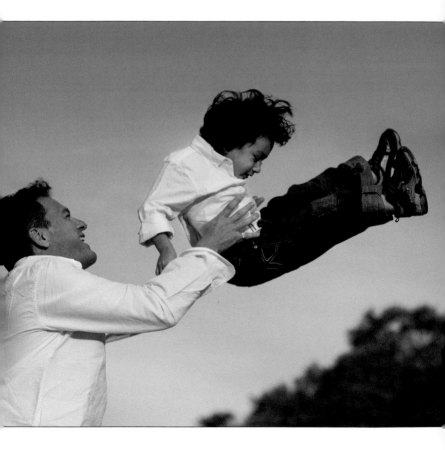

Fatherhood, for me, has been less a job than an
unstable and surprising combination of adventure'
blindman's bluff, guerrilla warfare, and crossword puzzle.
—FREDERIC F. VAN DE WATER

• •

Reasoning with a child is fine, if you can reach
the child's reason without destroying your own.
—JOHN MASON BROWN, QUOTED IN *THE BEST OF
FATHER QUOTATIONS,* ED. HELEN EXLEY (1995)

• • •

Children are a poor man's riches.
—ENGLISH PROVERB

• •

I can always count on getting one thing for Father's
Day—all the bills from Mother's Day.
—MILTON BERLE

• • •

Children of the new millennium when change is
likely to continue and stress will be inevitable,
are going to need, more than ever, the mentoring
of an available father.
—IAN GRANT, *FATHERS WHO DARE TO WIN (1999)*

• •

A Hard Profession

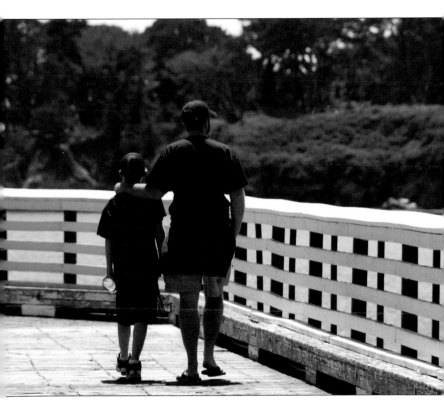

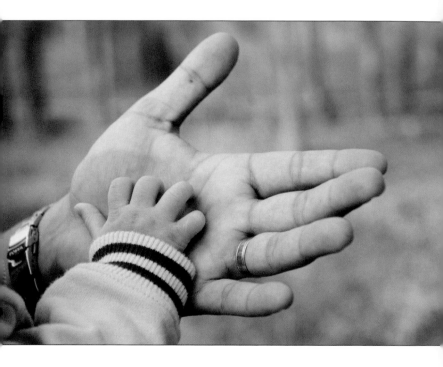

All I could see was that I was going to lose him,
just as my own father had lost me.
—WILLIAM PLUMMER, *WISHING
MY FATHER WELL (2000)*

• • •

Fatherhood has been known to transform even
the toughest and most resilient into a quivering mass.
—MARCUS JACOB GOLDMAN, *THE JOY OF
FATHERIIOOD (2000)*

• •

To be happy, fathers must always be giving; it is ceaselessly giving that makes you really a father.
—GORIOT, IN *PERE GORIOT* BY HONORE DE BALZAC

• • •

Life doesn't come with an instruction book—that's why we have fathers.
—H. JACKSON BROWNE'S DAD, AS QUOTED IN *A FATHER'S BOOK OF WISDOM (1988)*

• •

He felt that although his father loved their home and loved all of them, he was more lonely than the contentment of this family could help.
—JAMES AGEE

• • •

The worst misfortune that can happen to an ordinary
man is to have an extraordinary father.
—AUSTIN O'MALLEY

• •

This is the hardest truth for a father to learn: that
his children are continuously growing up and
moving away from him (until, of course, they
move back in).
—BILL COSBY, *FATHERHOOD*

• • •

No man is responsible for his father. That is entirely
his mother's affair.
—MARGARET TRUMBULL

• •

A king, realizing his incompetence, can either
delegate or abdicate his duties. A father can do
neither.
—MARLENE DIETRICH (QUOTED IN *DADS,*
JUNE/JULY 2000)

• • •

Setting a good example for children takes all the
fun out of middle age.
—WILLIAM FEATHER

• •

In America there are two classes of travel—first
class and with children.
—ROBERT BENCHLEY

• • •

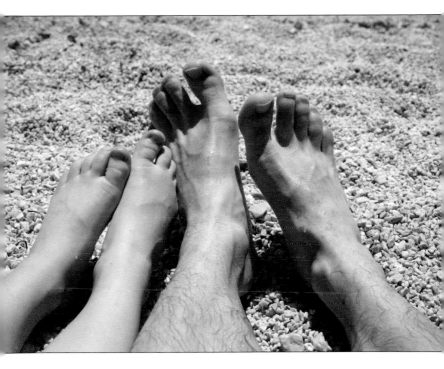

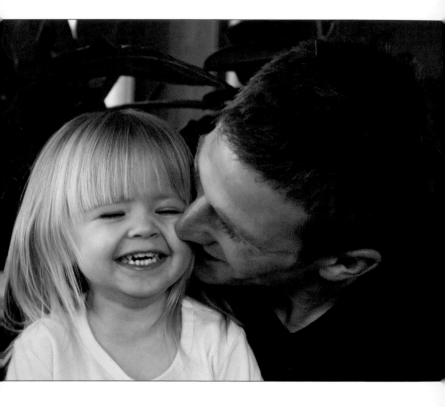

There are three ways to get something done:
(1) Do it yourself.
(2) Hire someone to do it for you.
(3) Forbid your kids to do it.
—AUTHOR UNKNOWN

• •

. . . if you see the challenge of fathering as the
biggest victory of your life, it will be a goal worth
stretching for.
—IAN GRANT, *FATHERS WHO DARE TO WIN (1999)*

• • •

Children today are tyrants. They contradict their
parents, gobble their food, and tyrannize their teachers.
—SOCRATES

• •

More than anything I had wanted to build a
sturdy bridge to my son before adolescence set
in. But I was afraid that instead I had merely
deepened the moat around him.
—WILLIAM PLUMMER, *WISHING MY
FATHER WELL (2000)*

• • •

PART SEVEN

Appreciating Dad

Directly after God in heaven comes papa.
—W. A. MOZART(1756–1791)

• • •

I watched a small man with thick calluses on
both hands work fifteen and sixteen hours a day.
I saw him once literally bleed from the bottom
of his feet, a man who came here uneducated,
alone, unable to speak the language, who taught
me all I needed to know about faith and hard
work by the simple eloquence of his example.
—MARIO CUOMO

• •

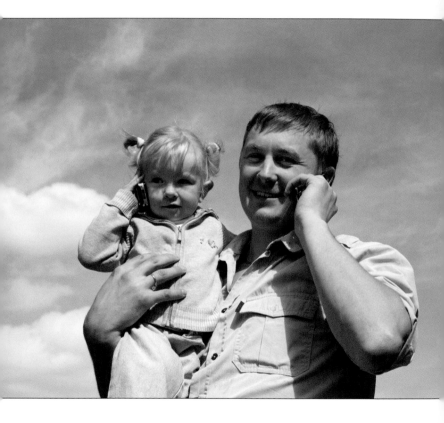

A father is a banker provided by nature.
—FRENCH PROVERB

• • •

How true daddy's words were when he said: "All children must look after their own upbringing."
—ANNE FRANK

• •

His values embraced family, reveled in the social mingling of the kitchen, and above all, welcomed the loving disorder of children.
—JOHN COLE

• • •

Be kind to thy father, for when thou wert young,
Who loved thee so fondly as he?
He caught the first accents that fell
from thy tongue,
And joined in thy innocent glee.
—MARGARET COURTNEY

• •

When one has not had a good father, one must
create one.
—FRIEDRICH NIETZSCHE

• • •

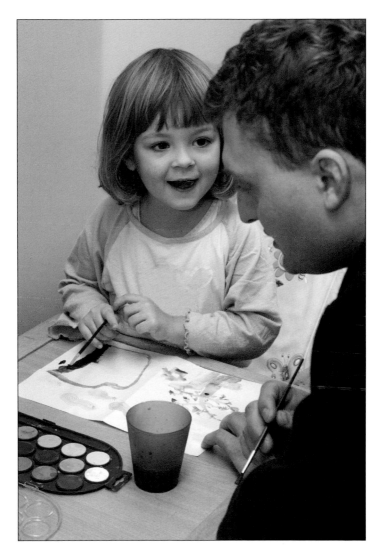

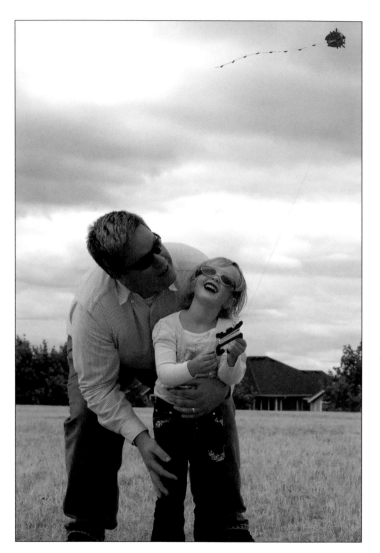

. . . my father studied cattle with the same fascination
with which I study books.
—LARRY McMURTRY, *WALTER BENJAMIN AT THE
DAIRY QUEEN (1999)*

• •

In the natural way of things, children only have a
father for a few brief moments.
—HONORE DE BALZAC, *THE GIRL WITH THE
GOLDEN EYES*

• • •

He is the stuff of which sitcoms are made.
—ANGELA CARTER,"SUGAR DADDY," *THE GRANTA
BOOK OF THE FAMILY (1995)*

• •

I talk and talk and talk, and I haven't taught
people in fifty years what my father taught by
example in one week.
—MARIO CUOMO

• • •

My father is my idol, so I always did everything
like him. He used to work two jobs and still come
home happy every night. He didn't do drugs or
drink, and he wouldn't let anyone smoke in his
house. Those are the rules I adopted, too.
—EARVIN "MAGIC" JOHNSON

• •

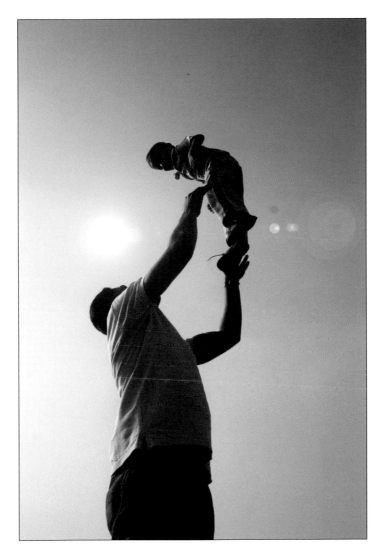

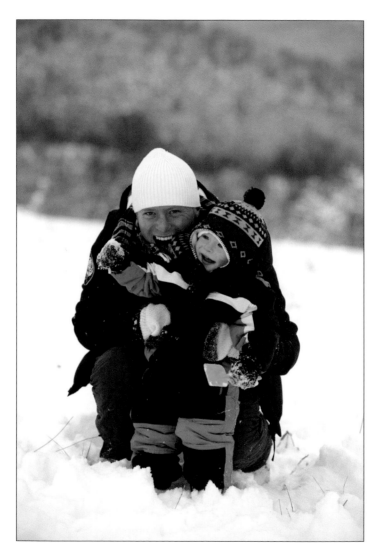

I have spent hours kicking myself for not fighting
past Dad's reserve, for not going into that
cave where he lived and rooting him out.
—WILLIAM PLUMMER, *WISHING MY
FATHER WELL (2000)*

• • •

'Tis happy for him, that his father was before him.
—JONATHAN SWIFT

• •

The search for a father is a search for authority
outside of yourself; you feel wraithlike, incomplete
without him, in whatever form he takes.
—NICK LYONS

• • •

When I was fourteen, my father was so ignorant
I could hardly stand to have the old man
around. But when I got to be twenty-one, I was
astonished at how much he had learned in
seven years.
—MARK TWAIN

• •

When he first thought about him it was always
the eyes . . . they saw much further and much
quicker than the human eye sees and they were
the great gift his father had. His father saw as a
bighorn ram or as an eagle sees, literally.
—ERNEST HEMINGWAY, "FATHERS AND SONS"

• • •

Appreciating Dad

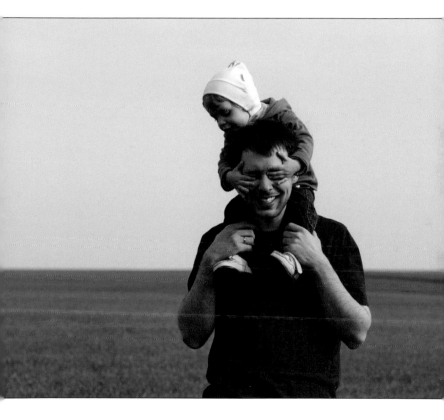

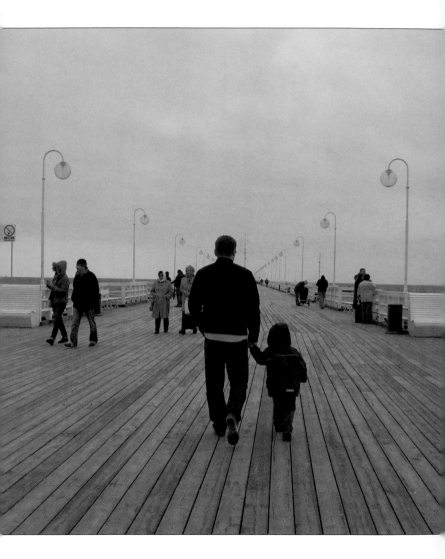

Middle Age
At forty-five,
What next, what next?
At every corner,
I meet my Father,
My age, still alive.
—ROBERT LOWELL

• •

My father was a statesman. I'm a political woman.
My father was a saint. I'm not.
—INDIRA GANDHI

• • •

You can't compare me to my father. Our similarities
are different.
—DALE BERRA, SON OF YOGI BERRA

• •

Some day you will know that a father is much
happier in his children's happiness than in his
own. I cannot explain it to you: it is a feeling in
your body that spreads gladness through you.
—HONORE DE BALZAC, *PERE GORIOT*

• • •

Appreciating Dad

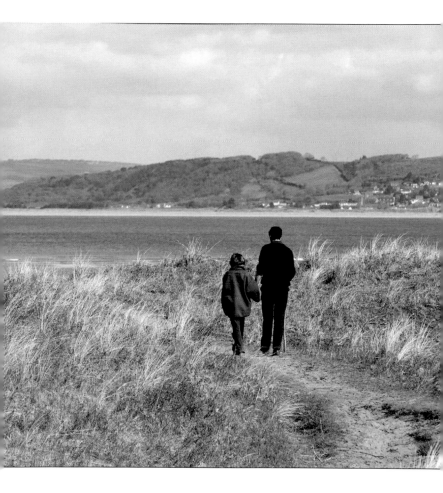

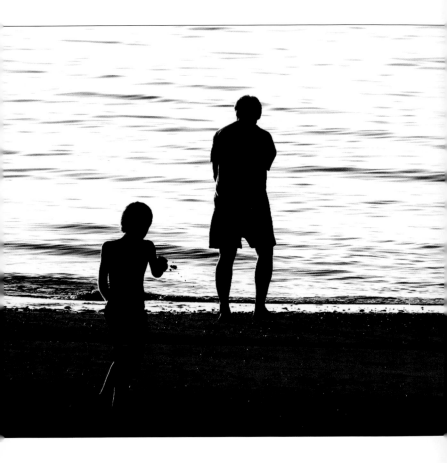

The greatest legacy a man can leave in the world
is not so much a great business, but a "living" investment
in the future, through loving, stable,
employable and healthy children.
—IAN GRANT, *FATHERS WHO DARE TO WIN (1999)*

• •

My father was not a failure. After all, he was the
father of a president of the United States.
—HARRY S TRUMAN

• • •

. . . it took me years to recognize my father's depths, how I am sounding them still. . . . All I ever saw, growing up, was his difference from me.
—WILLIAM PLUMMER, *WISHING MY FATHER WELL (2000)*

PART EIGHT

• •

The Later Years

The simplest toy, one which even the youngest
child can operate, is called a grandparent.
—SAM LEVENSON

• • •

By the time a man realizes that maybe his father
was right, he usually has a son who thinks he's
wrong.
—CHARLES WADSWORTH

• •

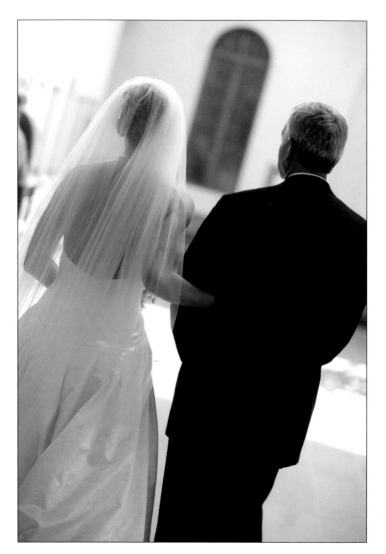

What you have inherited from your father, you
must earn over again for yourselves, or it will not
be yours.
—JOHANN WOLFGANG von GOETHE

• • •

A man knows when he is growing old because
he begins to look like his father.
—GABRIEL GARCIA MARQUEZ

• •

I suppose you think that persons who are as old
as your father and myself are always thinking
about very grave things, but I know that we are
meditating the same old themes that we did
when we were ten years old, only we go more
gravely about it.
—H. D. THOREAU, TO ELLEN EMERSON,
R. W. EMERSON'S DAUGHTER

• • •

My father died at 102. Whenever I would ask
what kept him going, he'd answer, "*I* never
worry."
—JERRY STILLER, *MARRIED TO LAUGHTER (2000)*

• •

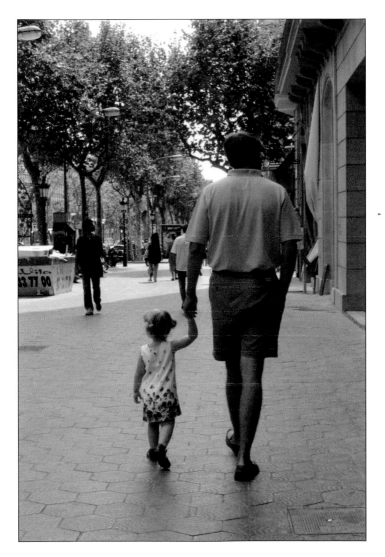

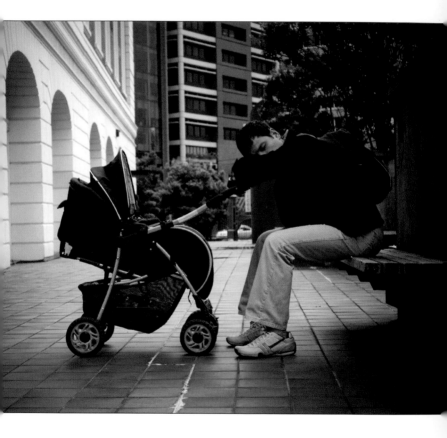

Nothing I've ever done has given me more joys
and rewards than being a father to my five.
—BILL COSBY, *FATHERHOOD*

• • •

In peace the sons bury their fathers, but in war
the fathers bury their sons.
—CROESUS

• •

And though I know we are different, I am grateful
for what I have of my father in me. It is my
gift, my promise to myself and my children.
—KENNETH BARRETT

• • •

... . my father's career and my own were not
as different as I had once thought. He cattle
ranched in a time he didn't like much, and I
word ranched.
—LARRY McMURTRY, *WALTER BENJAMIN AT THE
DAIRY QUEEN (1999)*

• •

Even though I hated him for dying and abandoning
me, I would go to a closet in the den and
take out photographs of my father when no one
was home. I would stare at them, searching for a
trace of myself, to see what I had that would
identify me as his son.
—DAVID SEYBOLD

• • •

By the time the youngest children have learned
to keep the house tidy, the oldest grandchildren
are on hand to take it to pieces.
—CHRISTOPHER MORLEY

• •

You feel completely comfortable entrusting your
baby to them for long periods, which is why
most grandparents flee to Florida at the earliest
opportunity.
—DAVE BARRY

• • •

My son and my father. Two sons, two fathers. Yet
three people. We walk behind a father's name,
shoulder a father's memory. Wear another's walk,
another's gait. Wait for what has happened to
their bodies, the same scars, maladies, aches, to
surface in ours.
—FRED D'AGUIAR, "A SON IN SHADOW"
(HARPER'S MAGAZINE, 1999)

• •

There are three stages of a man's life:
1. He believes in Santa Claus.
2. He doesn't believe in Santa Claus.
3. He is Santa Claus.
—AUTHOR UNKNOWN

• • •

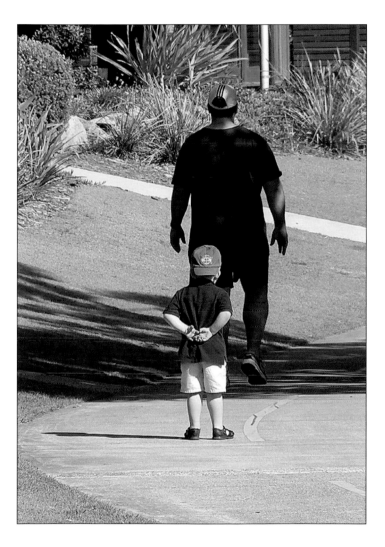

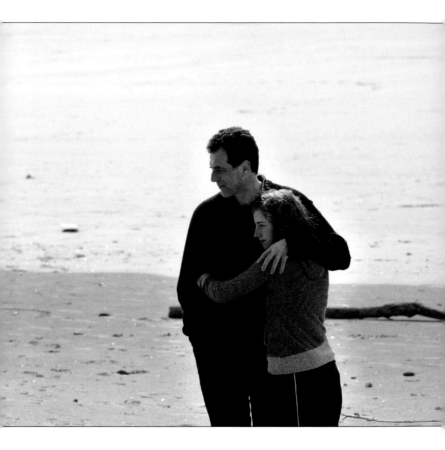

Every generation revolts against its fathers and
makes friends with its grandfathers.
—LEWIS MUMFORD

• •

There's one thing about children—they never go
around showing snapshots of their grandparents.
—LEOPOLD FECHTNER

• • •

Grandpa, you're the handsomest man in the
world, after my dad. And, Grandpa, you're the
best storyteller ever.
—LARA, AGED FIVE

• •

Grandparents range from infantile to mature,
like everybody else.
—JEAN MARZOLLO, *FATHERS AND BABIES (1993)*

• • •

When I was a boy I used to do what my father
wanted. Now I have to do what my boy wants. My
problem is: when I am going to do what I want.
—SAM LEVENSON

• •

One of life's greatest mysteries is how the boy
who wasn't good enough to marry your daughter
can be the father of the smartest grandchild
in the world.
—JEWISH PROVERB

• • •

A child enters your home and for the next
twenty years makes so much noise you can
hardly stand it. The child departs, leaving the
house so silent you think you are going mad.
—JOHN ANDREW HOLMES

• •

I kept thinking what a wonderful old man he
would have made if he had learned how, and
further, I didn't think he'd ever faced up to becoming old.
—JACK HEMINGWAY, OF HIS FATHER ERNEST, IN
MISADVENTURES OF A FLY FISHERMAN (1986)

• • •

My father always used to say that when you
die, if you've got five real friends, you've had a
great life.
—LEE IACOCCA

• •

He is tender and wary with his grandson, this
messenger of life and his mortality.
—MICHAEL IGNATIEFF, "AUGUST IN MY
FATHER'S HOUSE," *THE GRANTA BOOK OF THE
FAMILY (1995)*

• • •

You've got to do your own growing, no matter
how tall your grandfather was.
—IRISH PROVERB

• •

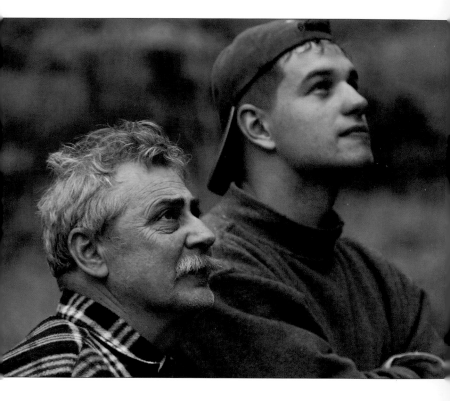

Dad and I never run out of things to talk about,
but I am content that he and I have said everything
that needs saying already. It's never been hard.
—WILLIAM G. TAPPLY, *SPORTSMAN'S LEGACY (1993)*

• • •

When you teach your son, you teach your son's
son.
—THE TALMUD

• •

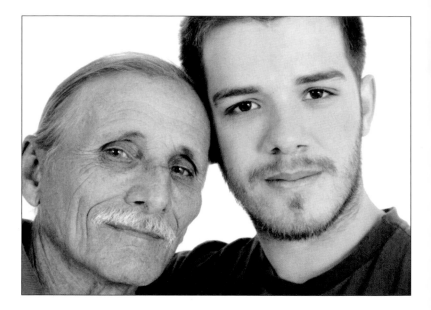

Index

Index

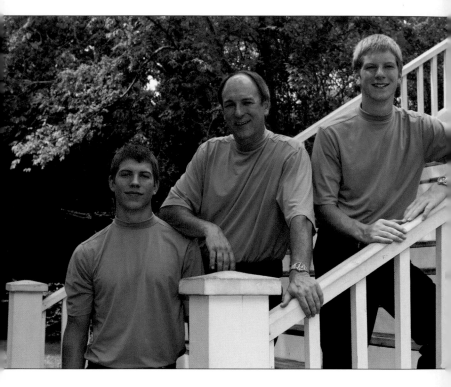